T0314549

SPORTS INJURIES:
THEIR TREATMENT
BY HOMOEOPATHY
AND ACUPRESSURE

by

LESLIE J. SPEIGHT

THE C. W. DANIEL COMPANY LIMITED
CHURCH PATH, SAFFRON WALDEN
ESSEX

First published in Great Britain by
The C. W. Daniel Company Limited
1 Church Path, Saffron Walden
Essex CB10 1JP, England

ISBN 0 85207 213 9

Reprinted May 1992

The Random House Group Limited supports The Forest Stewardship
Council (FSC®), the leading international forest certification organisation.
Our books carrying the FSC label are printed on FSC® certified paper.
FSC is the only forest certification scheme endorsed by the leading
environmental organisations, including Greenpeace. Our
paper procurement policy can be found at
www.randomhouse.co.uk/environment

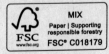

Printed and bound in Great Britain by Clays Ltd, St Ives PLC

Set by MS Typesetting, Castle Camps, Cambridge

CONTENTS

INTRODUCTION

This book is, to a large extent, an enlarged and revised edition of *Athletic Injuries* by Dr. P. H. Sharp which has been out of print for a considerable time.

The treatments recommended do not usurp the functions of trainers and those attendant on sport who know a great deal about the immediate treatment of injuries and who, as a rule, combine the best features of a doctor and a skilled osteopath.

In these days of intense competition in the athletic sphere, both amateur and professional, calling for extreme endeavour on the part of sportsmen (and sportswomen) there is an ever increasing number of injuries and in the case of professionals the financial rewards are such that trainers and others associated with the welfare of athletes are under extreme pressure to overcome the trouble in the shortest possible time; in fact one suspects that many athletes return to the fray before their injuries are completely healed — time is money!

Homoeopathic treatment does not supplant the manipulative therapy which is usually most helpful but homoeopathic remedies are usually speedier in action and more effective than the usual drug therapy. In addition, there is no risk of undesirable effects which can often occur after the administration of orthodox drugs.

1

Once the benefits of homoeopathic treatment are experienced there is no doubt that open-minded trainers and others will use the remedies in all suitable cases.

It can be fairly claimed that homoeopathy gives earlier relief from shock and pain, and quicker and more lasting healing of sprains, fractures and other injuries. The manipulations of the trainer based on the sound principle of restoring position and function at the earliest moment are not, of course, called into question. It will be found that homoeopathic treatments supplement them and provide speedy recovery.

It should not be thought that homoeopathy merely consists of picking a particular remedy for a particular complaint; the personal make-up and idiosyncrasies of the patient vary and these factors determine the selection of the remedy, although this happens less in the case of injuries such as are mentioned in this book, than is the case of illnesses.

Any attempt to introduce these variations would have converted into an exhaustive volume what is merely intended to be a brief introduction to the possibilities of homoeopathic treatment in sports injuries to those who have not previously considered its application in this direction.

In order to simplify the selection of the appropriate remedy only the principal ones are mentioned and as they are effective in a very high percentage of cases it is hoped that success will stimulate interest and lead to a desire for more knowledge of the subject, which can be obtained from the extensive literature now available.

SPORTS INJURIES AND CONDITIONS

Sports injuries are no different essentially from injuries arrived at in other ways, and if one is struck by a hockey stick, the results are pretty similar whether the assailant's intentions are felonious or sportive. Certain injuries and conditions, however, have a habit of cropping up in sport, and each particular sport has its own collection of regular injuries. To those engaged in these activities the problem is viewed from a different angle from that of the doctor.

The doctor in effect says: 'Here is an injury; certain damage has been done. We will do so-and-so, and modify the treatment from time to time as the occasion demands, and when the injury is quite healed, the patient may go about his business.'

This is quite sound, especially if we have plenty of time, but it would not satisfy the average football trainer who has to be doctor-on-the-spot and take quick hair-raising decisions without the protection of a medical degree behind him.

To those engaged in sport a series of questions immediately arise, following an injury, namely:-

(1) Can the player or contestant continue?
(2) What is the immediate treatment?
(3) What is the treatment following the game or contest?
(4) What is the period of disability?
(5) Can complete function be restored?

Good trainers (and few, if any, are bad) have these points always before them, and their answers in the main are good and practical. It is assumed, then, that if homoeopathy can offer them further worthwhile means of dealing with these problems, they will be willing and eager to accept them. It may be said now, with confidence, that homoeopathy can afford the greatest immediate relief; can give the following treatment which will ease pain while healing; and can considerably shorten the period of disability and hasten the good functional result.

Let us take three of our remedies out of turn to stress the above claims:—

SHOCK. All falls and knocks are accompanied by a varying degree of shock; a dose of homoeopathic *Arnica* of the correct strength, taken by mouth, will immediately ameliorate the shock and prevent its worst effects.

BLEEDING. A few drops of tincture of *Calendula* on a cut will almost immediately stop bleeding. It is not expected that boxing trainers will give up their Collodion, but they might try out *Calendula* in training before applying the Collodion.

FRACTURES. A fracture heals much quicker and with much less pain if the patient takes *Symphytum* for the first few days.

The above are just three examples of the really practical nature of this form of treatment, and the fact that it works every time will soon convince practical men of its usefulness.

It is proposed in this small book to take each sport separately and deal with its injuries and their treatment under that heading. This will necessarily involve a considerable degree of repetition as some injuries and their treatment are common to all sports. However, it has been considered to be the only practical arrangement which will facilitate quick reference to the sport and injury which is being sought.

It is not proposed to differentiate between professional and amateur sport; such a distinction would be quite artificial, and from the treatment angle all players go in the same door; consequently for the word 'trainer' one may substitute the word 'coach' or 'instructor'.

Finally only the principal sports are here considered, but these may be regarded as giving the full range of probable injuries and, in addition, a materia medica will list the range of remedies and briefly describe their uses; thus, should one sustain an injury while playing any other sport, it should be possible by studying an analogous sport and the materia medica, to decide on the appropriate treatment.

Let us then consider our sports, their injuries and their treatment, and see what homoeopathy has to offer which is good and practical.

TWO CASE HISTORIES

Here are two cases extracted from *Homoeopathy for the first-aider* by Dr. Dorothy Shepherd which illustrate the efficacy of homoeopathy.

'A lad of twelve, while riding on a high milk delivery cart, was pitched off and fell on his face, on the stone pavement. He had just time to whisper "take me to the Sister of the Mission, not to hospital" before he lost his senses. He was brought into the clinic suffering from shock, pale and cold, the pulse was irregular, the left side of his face was swollen and deep purple, his left eye was closed and swollen. He was given *Arnica* every 15 minutes and his face dressed with a *Calendula* dressing. After the first dose of *Arnica* he went to sleep; when I saw him two hours later his pulse and respiration were steady. The Sister stated that the swelling had already much improved as he had looked almost dead when carried into the surgery. He tried to sit up as I spoke to him and declared he felt much more himself, then he brought up some undigested food. Three hours after the accident he walked home looking greatly improved. He rested in bed for the rest of the day at his home, taking *Arnica*, 4 hourly. The swelling of the left cheek and eye was much diminished by the next morning when he walked, jauntily, into the surgery; the swelling of the face and eye cleared in under four days, and he was back at the milk round in time for the Saturday delivery. Surely a most satisfactory and rapid cure.

A similar case was that of a girl of about fourteen years of age who was brought in by her companions after a similar fall on the paving stones. Her features were unrecognizable, both eyes closed by the swelling. The face was a purple pulpy mass, blood streaming all over her. She was cleaned up with *Calendula* and a cold *Calendula* dressing was applied to the face. *Arnica* was given 2 hourly at first and then 4 hourly, within two days the face had almost returned to normal. There was no sepsis and she was discharged completely cured in five days.'

ABOUT HOMOEOPATHIC REMEDIES

To those with no knowledge of homoeopathy the preparation of the remedies is somewhat confusing. They are available in liquids, granules, pills and tablets, each being equally effective, and the prescriber should choose the form most suitable to his requirements. It is suggested that granules might be most suitable as two or three of these can be placed in the mouth (under the tongue is best) and they dissolve in a very short time.

A dose is 1 pill or tablet and 1 drop of a liquid except for mother tinctures (Ø) for which detailed instructions are given.

Always store homoeopathic remedies away from strong perfumes, camphor, peppermint etc., and in a dark, cool place.

It will be observed that the name of each remedy is followed by a number. This (called potency) indicates the strength of the medicine and in order to assist those without knowledge of homoeopathic prescribing we have suggested a suitable potency against each remedy. The remedies, however, can be used in other strengths with equally good results. For instance, if a 6 is recommended but only a 12 or 30 is available do not hesitate in using it but remember that the higher the number the deeper its action and it does not need to be prescribed so frequently.

Always procure homoeopathic remedies from a chemist specializing in this type of pharmacy as the medicines must be prepared from the correct ingredients and then potentised properly, a process that should be carried out only by those with experience in this method of pharmacy.

BEFORE THE EVENT

Sportsmen of all persuasions suffer some degree of apprehension, excitement, stress, etc., which manifests in a variety of symptoms according to the idiosyncracy of the individual.

ACUTE ANXIETY, RESTLESSNESS, FEARFULNESS, IMPATIENCE. *Aconite 30.*

APPREHENSION without any clear-cut symptoms. *Argentum Nitricum 30.*

APPREHENSION with EXCITEMENT, TREMBLING often accompanied by DIARRHOEA. Individual quiet and subdued. *Gelsemium 30.*

LACK OF CONFIDENCE. *Anacardium 30.*

SLEEPLESSNESS caused by over-active brain brought on by anticipation. *Coffea 200.* This potency is likely to be the most effective in this condition and a dose an hour before retiring and another at bedtime should be given. If the 200th is not available use the 30th in the same manner.

Generally give a dose of the remedy one hour before the event and a second immediately before the event.

Should the 6th or 12th potency be used an extra dose may be given half-an-hour before the event.

BOXING

It is necessary to distinguish between the immediate and the later treatment of injuries, and the trainer will have to decide upon the extent to which homoeopathic remedies should be administered during a contest — what is permissible as well as practical. To pop pills or drops into a contestant's mouth between rounds might excite justifiable curiosity on the part of the referee and lead to controversy although the remedies are not drugs and analysis could never detect any prohibited substance.

BLACK EYE. *Ledum 200* is almost a specific, especially if the pain is relieved by cold applications. Three doses should be given at four hourly intervals.

If there is no relief from cold applications *Staphisagria 200* should be given in the same dosages as for *Ledum*.

Remember that two black eyes administered simultaneously may indicate a fractured base of the skull.

BLEEDING. A few drops of *Calendula Ø* (mother tincture) applied to a wound will stop bleeding very quickly and a dose of *Arnica 30* (internally) will help to overcome any shock and enhance the healing process.

Should the *Calendula* fail to control the

bleeding give *Ferrum Phosphoricum 6* or *12* or *Vipera 12* (internally) every few minutes for a few doses. These remedies act promptly and usually stop bleeding very quickly. Use whichever remedy is available but Dr. Dorothy Shepherd seemed to consider *Vipera* the more effective.

Where the bleeding does not respond quickly, especially if the blood is bright red, give a dose or two of *Phosphorus 12* but seek professional assistance if the remedies fail to stop the bleeding within a reasonable time.

BRUISES. Of muscles and soft parts should be treated internally with *Arnica 30*, the first dose given as soon as possible after the injury and then at hourly intervals for three doses followed by a dose night and morning until the bruise has disappeared. This remedy will also help to overcome any shock.

Bruising of the bone and periosteum requires a dose of *Arnica 30* to allay the shock followed within a few minutes by *Ruta 30* at hourly intervals for three doses and then night and morning until the trouble has cleared.

Old bruises, often with discoloration and knots, are frequently cleared by *Sulphuric Acid 6* three times daily for a few weeks.

CONCUSSION. Any injury to the head must be accompanied by shock, so give a dose of *Arnica 30* immediately and then at half-hourly intervals for five or six doses.

In cases of Concussion of the Spine caused by a sudden fall on the base of the spine (Coccyx) a dose of *Arnica 30* followed by *Hypericum 30* within a few minutes and then at half-hourly intervals for five or six doses.

CRAMP. For contraction of the muscles and tendons give one or two doses of *Cuprum 12* or

30 at ten minute intervals. *Ledum 12* or *30* in the same dosage is another effective remedy. When fatigue is the cause *Arnica 30* should be given in the same dosage.

CRUSHED FINGERS, TOES, COCCYX (base of spine) and other parts rich in nerve endings. Give a dose of *Arnica 30* immediately to counteract the shock and follow within ten minutes with *Hypericum 30* every fifteen minutes but extend the time between doses as the pain recedes.

CUTS. *Calendula Ø* applied immediately will usually check the bleeding and also inhibit the growth of bacteria and prevent infection. The seconds may feel impelled to apply flexible Collodion (or some other substance) above this to enable the boxer to carry on with the contest but the *Calendula* will greatly speed the healing and the cut should be bathed with one part of *Calendula Ø* to ten of water at intervals until the wound has healed, this will help to strengthen the skin and enable it to withstand subsequent blows with less risk of damage. *Calendula 30* taken internally three times daily for two or three days will supplement the healing process and lead to even quicker results.

EYEBALL. If a blow has caused it to be very tender and water *Hypericum 30* at four hourly intervals for a few doses.

HEART. A blow over the heart often causes great pain and a feeling as though the heart were gripped in a vice. A dose of *Arnica 30* to combat the shock followed by *Cactus 12* every fifteen minutes until the pain is eased.

NOSE BLEED. A plug soaked in *Calendula Ø* will stop bleeding very quickly but if the spot cannot be reached give *Arnica 12* every few minutes until improvement sets in and then less frequently. Two other remedies which are very effective in checking bleeding, when taken internally, are *Ferrum Phosphoricum 12* and *Vipera 12* every few minutes until the bleeding has stopped. Dr. Dorothy Shepherd seemed to believe that *Vipera* is the more effective remedy.

Where bleeding does not respond quickly, especially if the blood is bright red, *Phosphorus 12* for dose or two but seek professional assistance if the remedies fail to bring the bleeding under control quickly.

TORN MUSCLES. Often the result of excessive strain, respond to *Agaricus 6* night and morning for a week or two.
Where injury makes the patient incapable of movement *Bryonia 30* every half-an-hour for three doses and then night and morning for a few days, if necessary.

CRICKET

BLEEDING. A few drops of *Calendula Ø* (mother tincture) applied to a wound will stop bleeding very quickly and a dose of *Arnica 30* (internally) will help to overcome any shock and enhance the healing process.

Should the *Calendula* fail to control the bleeding give *Ferrum Phosphoricum 6* or *12* or *Vipera 12* (internally) every few minutes for a few doses. These remedies act promptly and usually stop bleeding very quickly. Use whichever remedy is available but Dr. Dorothy Shepherd seemed to consider *Vipera* the more effective.

Where the bleeding does not respond quickly, especially if the blood is bright red, give a dose or two of *Phosphorus 12* but seek professional assistance if the remedies fail to stop the bleeding within a reasonable time.

BRUISES. Of muscles and soft parts should be treated internally with *Arnica 30*, the first dose given as soon as possible after the injury and then at hourly intervals for three doses followed by a dose night and morning until the bruise has disappeared. This remedy will also help to overcome any shock.

Bruising of the bone and periosteum requires a dose of *Arnica 30* to allay the shock followed within a few minutes by *Ruta 30* at hourly intervals for three doses and then night and morning until the trouble has cleared.

Old bruises, often with discoloration and knots, are frequently cleared by *Sulphuric Acid 6* three times daily for a few weeks.

CONCUSSION. Any injury to the head must be accompanied by shock, so give a dose of *Arnica 30* immediately and then at half-hourly intervals for five or six doses.

In cases of Concussion of the Spine caused by a sudden fall on the base of the spine (Coccyx) a dose of *Arnica 30* followed by *Hypericum 30* within a few minutes and then at half-hourly intervals for five or six doses.

CRAMP. For contraction of the muscles and tendons give one or two doses of *Cuprum 12* or *30* at ten-minute intervals. *Ledum 12* or *30* in the same dosage is another effective remedy. When fatigue is the cause *Arnica 30* should be given in the same dosage.

CRUSHED FINGERS, TOES, COCCYX (base of spine) and other parts rich in nerve endings. Give a dose of *Arnica 30* immediately to counteract the shock and follow within ten minutes with *Hypericum 30* every fifteen minutes but extend the time between doses as the pain recedes.

CUTS. *Calendula Ø* (mother tincture) applied immediately will usually check bleeding, inhibit the growth of bacteria and prevent infection. *Calendula 30* taken internally three times daily for two or three days will supplement the healing process and lead to even quicker results.

FRACTURES. After the usual mechanical adjustment and, if necessary, splinting give *Symphytum 30* night and morning for about a week, this will bring about rapid union of the bones.

SPRAINS. Involving stretching of ligaments and tendons should be treated with *Rhus Toxicodendron 6* or *12* three times daily. This remedy is prescribed for rheumatism when the joints are worse in cold damp weather and as there is always the possibility of this trouble developing in an injured joint, *Rhus Toxicodendron* could abort it. If the rheumatism is better in cold damp weather give *Ledum 30* three times daily until better.

STRAINS. Involving wrenched muscles respond to *Arnica 12* three times daily for a few doses, but as there is always a degree of shock in these injuries one dose of Arnica 30 could be given before commencing with the lower potency.

Old strains associated with intermittent pains, swellings, easy relapses, can be helped by *Strontium Carbonicum 30* night and morning for a week or two.

SUNSTROKE. The usual first-aid measures should be applied immediately and the patient placed in the care of a doctor.

All clothing should be loosened or discarded and the patient placed in the horizontal position in a cool place. The cooling should not be too rapid but the entire body wiped with water or alcohol and then gently fanned. *Belladonna 30* will help if the pupils are dilated, the pulse bounding, the skin burning hot and dry; delirium may develop. Suggested dose: at half-hourly intervals for up to three doses and then less often.

Glonoine 30 is the remedy if there is throbbing, bursting headache, flushed face and sweaty skin. Dose: at half-hourly intervals for up to three doses and then less often.

TORN MUSCLES. Often the result of excessive strain, respond to *Agaricus 6* night and morning for a week or two.

Where injury makes the patient incapable of movement *Bryonia 30* every half-an-hour for three doses and then night and morning for a few days, if necessary.

FOOTBALL

The homoeopathic remedies recommended for injuries sustained on the football field are not to be regarded as supplanting the very efficient manipulative measures used by most trainers who combine great skill coupled with common sense and a practical knowledge of mechanics as applied to joints. Nevertheless, these remedies can reinforce such treatment and considerably speed recovery.

BLEEDING. A few drops of *Calendula Ø* (mother tincture) applied to a wound will stop bleeding very quickly and a dose of *Arnica 30* (internally) will help to overcome any shock and enhance the healing process.

Should the *Calendula* fail to control the bleeding give *Ferrum Phosphoricum 6* or *12* or *Vipera 12* (internally) every few minutes for a few doses. These remedies act promptly and usually stop bleeding very quickly. Use whichever remedy is available but Dr. Dorothy Shepherd seemed to consider *Vipera* the more effective.

Where the bleeding does not respond quickly, especially if the blood is bright red, give a dose or two of *Phosphorus 12* but seek professional assistance if the remedies fail to stop the bleeding within a reasonable time.

BRUISES. Of muscles and soft parts should be

treated internally with *Arnica 30*, the first dose given as soon as possible after the injury and then at hourly intervals for three doses followed by a dose night and morning until the bruise has disappeared. This remedy will also help to overcome any shock.

Bruising of the bone and periosteum requires a dose of *Arnica 30* to allay the shock followed within a few minutes by *Ruta 30* at hourly intervals for three doses and then night and morning until the trouble has cleared.

Old bruises, often with discoloration and knots, are frequently cleared by *Sulphuric Acid 6* three times daily for a few weeks.

CONCUSSION. Any injury to the head must be accompanied by shock, so give a dose of *Arnica 30* immediately and then at half-hourly intervals for five or six doses.

In cases of concussion of the spine caused by a sudden fall on the base of the spine (coccyx) a dose of *Arnica 30* followed by *Hypericum 30* within a few minutes and then at half-hourly intervals for five or six doses.

DISLOCATIONS. After reduction a dose of *Arnica 30* followed by *Rhus Toxicodendron 30* night and morning for a few days.

FRACTURES OR A TORN SEMILUNAR CARTILAGE. Will heal more rapidly and with much less pain if *Symphytum 30* is given night and morning for about a week.

NOSE BLEED. A plug soaked in *Calendula Ø* will stop bleeding very quickly but if the spot cannot be reached give *Arnica 12* every few minutes until improvement sets in and then less frequently. Two other remedies which are very effective in checking bleeding, when taken internally, are *Ferrum Phosphoricum 12* and

Vipera 12 every few minutes until the bleeding has stopped. Dr. Dorothy Shepherd seemed to believe that *Vipera* is the more effective remedy.

Where bleeding does not respond quickly, especially if the blood is bright red, *Phosphorus 12* for a dose or two but seek professional assistance if the remedies fail to bring the bleeding under control quickly.

SPRAINS. Involving stretching of ligaments and tendons should be treated with *Rhus Toxicodendron 6* or *12* three times daily. This remedy is prescribed for rheumatism when the joints are worse in cold damp weather and as there is always the possibility of this trouble developing in an injured joint, *Rhus Toxicodendron* could abort it. If the rheumatism is better in cold damp weather give *Ledum 30* three times daily until better.

STRAINS. Involving wrenched muscles respond to *Arnica 12* three times daily for a few doses, but as there is always a degree of shock in these injuries one dose of *Arnica 30* could be given before commencing with the lower potency.

Old strains associated with intermittent pains, swellings, easy relapses, can be helped by *Strontium Carbonicum 30* night and morning for a week or two.

SYNOVITIS. Often occurs after a sprain and *Rhus Toxicodendron 6* or *12* three times daily for a week or two has helped numerous sufferers. Where the trouble is associated with bruised bone and periosteum *Ruta 6* or *12* three times daily for a week or two is the remedy.

TENOSYNOVITIS. *Anacardium 200* night and morning for a few days will soothe the inflammation.

TORN MUSCLES. Often the result of excessive strain, respond to *Agaricus 6* night and morning for a week or two.

Where the injury makes the patient incapable of movement *Bryonia 30* every half-an-hour for three doses and then night and morning for a few days, if necessary.

NOTE: After a wound, sprain or fracture when a sufferer says 'Since my accident I sleep badly' one dose of Sticta Pulmonaria 200 *is often helpful.*

HOCKEY AND LACROSSE

BRUISES. Of muscles and soft parts should be treated internally with *Arnica 30*, the first dose given as soon as possible after the injury and then at hourly intervals for three doses followed by a dose night and morning until the bruise has disappeared. This remedy will also help to overcome any shock.

Bruising of the bone and periosteum requires a dose of *Arnica 30* to allay the shock followed within a few minutes by *Ruta 30* at hourly intervals for three doses and then night and morning until the trouble has cleared.

Old bruises, often with discoloration and knots, are frequently cleared by *Sulphuric Acid 6* three times daily for a few weeks.

CUTS. *Calendula Ø* (mother tincture) applied immediately will usually check bleeding, inhibit the growth of bacteria and prevent infection. *Calendula 30* taken internally three times daily for two or three days will supplement the healing process and lead to even quicker results.

SPRAINS. Involving stretching of ligaments and tendons should be treated with *Rhus Toxicodendron 6* or *12* three times daily. This remedy is prescribed for rheumatism when the joints are worse in cold damp weather and as there is always the possibility of this trouble developing in an injured joint, *Rhus Toxicodendron* could abort it. If the rheumatism is better in cold damp weather give *Ledum 30* three times daily until better.

STRAINS. Involving wrenched muscles respond to *Arnica 12* three times daily for a few doses, but as there is always a degree of shock in these injuries one dose of *Arnica 30* could be given before commencing with the lower potency. Old strains associated with intermittent pains, swellings, easy relapses, can be helped by *Strontium Carbonicum 30* night and morning for a week or two.

ICE HOCKEY

BRUISES. Of muscles and soft parts should be treated internally with *Arnica 30*, the first dose given as soon as possible after the injury and then at hourly intervals for three doses followed by a dose night and morning until the bruise has disappeared. This remedy will also help to overcome any shocks.

Bruising of the bone and periosteum requires a dose of *Arnica 30* to allay the shock followed within a few minutes by *Ruta 30* at hourly intervals for three doses and then night and morning until the trouble has cleared.

Old bruises, often with discoloration and knots, are frequently cleared by *Sulphuric Acid 6* three times daily for a few weeks.

CUTS. *Calendula Ø* (mother tincture) applied immediately will usually check bleeding, inhibit the growth of bacteria and prevent infection. *Calendula 30* taken internally three times daily for two or three days will supplement the healing process and lead to even quicker results.

FATIGUE. A dose of *Arnica 30* will give speedy relief.

A hot bath to which about 20 drops of *Arnica Ø* have been added is very soothing. This is also helpful as a footbath for tired and aching feet.

SPRAINS. Involving stretching of ligaments and tendons should be treated with *Rhus Toxicodendron 6* or *12* three times daily. This remedy is prescribed for rheumatism when the joints are worse in cold damp weather and as there is always the possibility of this trouble developing in an injured joint, *Rhus Toxicodendron* could abort it. If the rheumatism is better in cold damp weather give *Ledum 30* three times daily until better.

STRAINS. Involving wrenched muscles respond to *Arnica 12* three times daily for a few doses, but as there is always a degree of shock in these injuries one dose of *Arnica 30* could be given before commencing with the lower potency.

Old strains associated with intermittent pains, swellings, easy relapses, can be helped by *Strontium Carbonicum 30* night and morning for a week or two.

CONCUSSION. Any injury to the head must be accompanied by shock, so give a dose of *Arnica 30* immediately and then at half-hourly intervals for five or six doses.

In cases of concussion of the spine caused by a sudden fall on the base of the spine (coccyx) a dose of *Arnica 30* followed by *Hypericum 30* within a few minutes and then at half-hourly intervals for five or six doses.

RUGBY

BRUISES. Of mucles and soft parts should be treated internally with *Arnica 30*, the first dose given as soon as possible after the injury and then at hourly intervals for three doses followed by a dose night and morning until the bruise has disappeared. This remedy will also help to overcome any shock.

Bruising of the bone and periosteum requires a dose of *Arnica 30* to allay the shock followed within a few minutes by *Ruta 30* at hourly intervals for three doses and then night and morning until the trouble has cleared.

Old bruises, often with discoloration and knots, are frequently cleared by *Sulphuric Acid 6* three times daily for a few weeks.

CUTS. *Calendula Ø* (mother tincture) applied immediately will usually check bleeding, inhibit the growth of bacteria and prevent infection. *Calendula 30* taken internally three times daily for two or three days will supplement the healing process and lead to even quicker results.

FATIGUE. A dose of *Arnica 30* will give speedy relief.

A hot bath to which about 20 drops of *Arnica Ø* have been added is very soothing. This is also helpful as a footbath for tired and aching feet.

SPRAINS. Involving stretching of ligaments and tendons should be treated with *Rhus Toxicodendron 6* or *12* three times daily. This remedy is prescribed for rheumatism when the joints are worse in cold damp weather and as there is always the possibility of this trouble developing in an injured joint, *Rhus Toxicodendron* could abort it. If the rheumatism is better in cold damp weather give *Ledum 30* three times daily until better.

STRAINS. Involving wrenched muscles respond to *Arnica 12* three times daily for a few doses, but as there is always a degree of shock in these injuries one dose of *Arnica 30* could be given before commencing with the lower potency.

Old strains associated with intermittent pains, swellings, easy relapses, can be helped by *Strontium Carbonicum 30* night and morning for a week or two.

CONCUSSION. Any injury to the head must be accompanied by shock, so give a dose of *Arnica 30* immediately and then at half-hourly intervals for five or six doses.

In cases of concussion of the spine caused by a sudden fall on the base of the spine (coccyx) a dose of *Arnica 30* followed by *Hypericum 30* within a few minutes and then at half-hourly intervals for five or six doses.

RUNNING

BLEEDING. A few drops of *Calendula Ø* (mother tincture) applied to a wound will stop bleeding very quickly and a dose of *Arnica 30* (internally) will help to overcome any shock and enhance the healing process.

Should the *Calendula* fail to control the bleeding give *Ferrum Phosphoricum 6* or *12* or *Vipera 12* (internally) every few minutes for a few doses. These remedies act promptly and usually stop bleeding very quickly. Use whichever remedy is available but Dr. Dorothy Shepherd seemed to consider *Vipera* the more effective.

Where the bleeding does not respond quickly, especially if the blood is bright red, give a dose or two of *Phosphorus 12* but seek professional assistance if the remedies fail to stop the bleeding within a reasonable time.

BLISTERS. Apply *Calendula ointment* and give *Causticum 30* internally night and morning for two or three days.

BRUISES. Of muscles and soft parts should be treated internally with *Arnica 30*, the first dose given as soon as possible after the injury and then at hourly intervals for three doses followed by a dose night and morning until the bruise has disappeared. This remedy will also help to overcome any shock.

Bruising of the bone and periosteum requires a dose of *Arnica 30* to allay the shock followed within a few minutes by *Ruta 30* at hourly intervals for three doses and then night and morning until the trouble has cleared.

Old bruises, often with discoloration and knots, are frequently cleared by *Sulphuric Acid 6* three times daily for a few weeks.

CRAMP. For contraction of the muscles and tendons give one or two doses of *Cuprum 12* or *30* at ten-minute intervals. *Ledum 12* or *30* in the same dosage is another effective remedy.

When fatigue is the cause *Arnica 30* should be given in the same dosage.

FATIGUE. A dose of *Arnica 30* will give speedy relief.

A hot bath to which about 20 drops of *Arnica Ø* have been added is very soothing. This is also helpful as a footbath for tired and aching feet.

FOOT INJURIES. If there is any suppuration or they are healing badly *Silica 30* night and morning for three days.

SPIKING. A few drops of *Calendula Ø* (mother tincture) applied to the wound will stop bleeding very quickly, inhibit the growth of bacteria and overcome the risk of sepsis. A dose of *Arnica 30* (internally) will deal with any shock and enhance the healing process.

The wound should be covered by a pad soaked in one part of *Calendula Ø* (mother tincture) to ten parts of water which should be kept damp by pouring the liquid over the pad as soon as it dries.

Where bleeding is slow and the injured part white, puffy and cold give *Ledum 30* every hour for up to six doses.

In profuse haemorrhage of dark venous

blood give *Crotalus Horridus 30* at hourly intervals for up to six doses.

STITCH. A condition which is a grave handicap to many runners and it is usually difficult to deal with. *Agaricus 6* night and morning for a week or two will often reduce the tendency to attacks.

There is, however, a form of stitch which, when it comes on, renders the runner incapable of movement and any attempt to move makes the pain much worse. This form of stitch, which will obviously have put the runner out of the race, should be treated with *Bryonia 30*, a dose every half-an-hour until the pain is relieved.

TORN MUSCLES. Often the result of excessive strain, respond to *Agaricus 6* night and morning for a week or two.

Where the injury makes the patient incapable of movement *Bryonia 30* every half-an-hour for three doses and then night and morning for a few days, if necessary.

SWIMMING

CRAMP. For contraction of the muscles and tendons give one or two doses of *Cuprum 12* or *30* at ten-minute intervals. *Ledum 12* or *30* in the same dosage is another very effective remedy.

Swimmers subject to this trouble should take *Cuprum 30* night and morning for two days before a swim and a dose before commencing the swim. In many cases this will act as a preventative.

Where cramp is caused by fatigue take *Arnica 30*, two doses at ten-minute intervals.

EXHAUSTION. Long distance swimmers often suffer exhaustion and a dose of *Arnica 30* will do much to restore normality. An additional aid is a hot bath to which about 20 drops of *Arnica Ø* have been added, it is very comforting.

SEA SICKNESS. Often affects long-distance swimmers when the sea is rough. There are two main types. The first is the clammy type with cold sweat and a frequent inclination to swallow saliva; *Tabacum 12* taken at half-hourly intervals will generally bring about a good response.

The second type has great nausea, vertigo, faintness and sudden loss of orientation; *Cocculus Indicus 12* at half-hourly intervals is an effective remedy. Experienced swimmers will know their type and three doses of the indicated remedy taken at hourly intervals, the last just before starting the swim, should act as a preventative.

TENNIS

BRUISES. Of muscles and soft parts should be treated internally with *Arnica 30*, the first dose given as soon as possible after the injury and then at hourly intervals for three doses followed by a dose night and morning until the bruise has disappeared. This remedy will also help to overcome any shock.

Bruising of the bone and periosteum requires a dose of *Arnica 30* to allay the shock followed within a few minutes by *Ruta 30* at hourly intervals for three doses and then night and morning until the trouble has cleared.

Old bruises, often with discoloration and knots, are frequently cleared by *Sulphuric Acid 6* three times daily for a few weeks.

FATIGUE. A dose of *Arnica 30* will give speedy relief.

A hot bath to which about 20 drops of *Arnica Ø* have been added is very soothing. This is also helpful as a footbath for tired and aching feet.

SPRAINS. Involving stretching of ligaments and tendons should be treated with *Rhus Toxicodendron 6* or *12* three times daily. This remedy is prescribed for rheumatism when the joints are worse in cold damp weather and as there is always the possibility of this trouble developing in an injured joint, *Rhus Toxicoden-*

dron could abort it. If the rheumatism is better in cold damp weather give *Ledum 30* three times daily until better.

STRAINS. Involving wrenched muscles respond to *Arnica 12* three times daily for a few doses, but as there is always a degree of shock in these injuries one dose of *Arnica 30* could be given before commencing with the lower potency.

Old strains associated with intermittent pains, swellings, easy relapses, can be helped by *Strontium Carbonicum 30* night and morning for a week or two.

SUNSTROKE. The usual first-aid measures should be applied immediately and the patient placed in the care of a doctor.

All clothing should be loosened or discarded and the patient placed in the horizontal position in a cool place. The cooling should not be too rapid but the entire body wiped with water or alcohol and then gently fanned. *Belladonna 30* will help if the pupils are dilated, the pulse bounding, the skin burning hot and dry; delirium may develop. Suggested dose: at half-hourly intervals for up to three doses and then less often.

Glonoine 30 is the remedy if there is throbbing, bursting headache, flushed face and sweaty skin. Dose: at half-hourly intervals for up to three doses and then less often.

TENNIS ELBOW. Can be eased and even checked in the early stages by *Agaricus 6* three times daily for a week or two.

EXPLANATION OF THE MATERIA MEDICA

This materia medica provides additional information about the remedies recommended under each sport.

The characteristics and modalities of each remedy are clearly stated and where there is doubt about the selection of a remedy reference to this materia medica will clarify its action and help in selecting the one most suitable for the particular case.

Modalities are conditions which modify symptoms, in other words symptoms of 'aches and pains' would be found under many remedies but 'aches and pains which are better movement' would bring *Rhus Toxicodendron* mind and 'aches and pains worse movement' would indicate Bryonia.

A study of the materia medica will reveal that homoeopathic remedies can be used in a much wider field than is shown in this work and, hopefully, it will lead to a greater knowledge and understanding of the remedies for use in both the sporting and domestic spheres.

MATERIA MEDICA

ACONITE

Great fear and anxiety which accompany every ailment.
Forebodings, fears death and the future.
Weakness of mind and body leading to physical exhaustion.
Worse: Dry, cold winds which often bring on complaints; warm room; evening and night; lying on affected side.
Better: Open air.

AGARICUS

Jerking, twitching, trembling, itching.
Injuries to torn muscles caused by excessive strain.
Sensation as if pierced by a needle of ice.
Symptoms appear diagonally — as right arm and left leg.
Worse: Open, cold air; cold weather; before a thunderstorm; after eating.
Better: Moving about slowly.

ANACARDIUM

Excessive nervousness; anxiety; lack of self-confidence; funk.

Sensation of plug in various parts.
Worse: Application of hot water.
Better: Eating temporarily relieves all discomfort; when lying on side; from rubbing.

ARGENTUM NITRICUM

A great remedy for anticipation.
Apprehensive, fearful, anxious, nervous, impulsive, must walk fast, and wants to do all things in a hurry, time passes too slowly.
Loathes heights.
Great desire for sweets.
Intolerance of heat.
Worse: Warmth of any kind; at night; sweets; after eating; from emotions; left-side.
Better: Fresh air; cold; eructations; pressure.

ARNICA

Any symptoms resulting from trauma, e.g. concussion, headache of long standing, inflammation of eyes, deafness, etc.
Recent and remote affections from injuries especially contusion or blows.
Head alone or face alone hot, rest of body cool.
Sore aching, bruised feeling.
Everything on which he lies feels too hard.
Fears being touched by those coming towards him.
Worse: Least touch; motion; damp cold.
Better: Lying down or with head low.

BRYONIA

This patient is worse from the slightest motion. Even moving the eyes when very ill makes him feel worse.
Pains are tearing, stitching, worse movement.

Very irritable, will snap very quickly.
Dryness of mucous membranes from lips to rectum.
Faintness when sitting up in bed.
Great sense of insecurity, therefore anxious.
Excessive thirst for large amounts at long intervals.
Worse: Motion; touch; warmth; hot weather.
Better: Pressure; lying on painful side; rest; cold things.

COCCULUS

A leading remedy for seasickness.
Nausea with faintness and vomiting.
Aversion to food.
Vertigo on rising.
Worse: Eating; open air; smoking; swimming; noise; jar; after loss of sleep.

COFFEA

Great activity of mind and body with sleeplessness; restless; great sensitivity.
Troubles from sudden surprises.
Very sensitive to pain.
Worse: Excessive emotions; strong odours; noise; open air; cold; at night.
Better: Warmth; from lying down.

CROTALUS HORRIDUS

Has a deep action on the blood.
Haemorrhages of dark venous blood that does not clot.
Tendency to carbuncles.
Haemorrhage diathesis.
Worse: Right side; from a jar; on waking; open air; damp and wet.

CUPRUM

Spasmodic affections, cramps.
Mental and bodily exhaustion from over-exertion of mind or loss of sleep.
Jerking and twitching of muscles in extremities.
Worse: Vomiting; contact.
Better: During perspiration; drinking cold water.

FERRUM PHOSPHORICUM

Haemorrhages including nose bleed — blood bright red.
Early stages of a cold.
Frontal headache followed and relieved by nose bleed.
Worse: Touch; jar; motion; right side; night; 4 to 6 a.m.
Better: Cold applications.

GELSEMIUM

Dizziness, drowsiness, dullness, trembling.
Muscular weakness.
Apathy regarding illness.
General prostration.
Emotional excitement, apprehension, fright.
Diarrhoea from emotional excitement.
(An excellent flu remedy when chills run up and down the spine, muscular soreness and great prostration.)
Worse: Damp weather; before a thunderstorm; emotion or excitement; bad news; tobacco smoke.
Better: Bending forward; open air; continued motion; copious urination relieves headaches.

GLONOINE

Sensation of pulsation throughout the body.
Pulsating pains.

Confusion in head with dizziness, cannot bear heat around head.
Throbbing.
Worse: Exposure to the sun; gas or open fire; stooping; having hair cut; lying down; from 6 a.m., until noon; left side.
Better: Brandy.

HYPERICUM

The great remedy for injuries to nerves; toes, fingers, coccyx (base of spine) and all parts rich in nerves.
Excessive painfulness.
Puncture wounds from nails, splinters, pins, stings, bites etc.
Relieves pain after operations.
Concussion of spine.
Prevents lockjaw if pains travel up limb away from the wound.
Worse: In cold; dampness; fog; closed room; least exposure; touch.
Better: Bending head backwards.

LEDUM

Puncture wounds from sharp-pointed instruments — nails, needles, bites etc., especially where there is little bleeding and part is cold, puffy and pale. If tetanus is threatened with these symptoms and there is twitching of muscles near the wound Ledum will clear up the trouble.
Bites of animals — dogs, rats etc.
Almost a specific for black eye.
Cramp.
Worse: At night; from heat of bed.
Better: From cold; cold water; putting feet in cold water gives relief.

41

PHOSPHORUS

Extremely sensitive and very fearful; of the dark; of thunderstorms; disease; death, etc.
Very affectionate.
Pains are burning.
Haemorrhages bright red and flowing freely.
Thirst for cold drinks which are vomited as soon as they get warm in the stomach.
Worse: Physical or mental exertion; touch; twilight; warm food or drink; from getting wet in hot weather; change of weather; lying on painful side.
Better: Heat (everywhere except stomach and head).

RHUS TOXICODENDRON

A remedy for sprains, acting on the fibrous and muscular tissues — joints, tendons, sheaths.
Hot painful swelling of joints.
Tearing pains in tendons and ligaments.
Rheumatism, lumbago, pains aggravated by cold and damp conditions.
Sitting or lying in one position causes stiffness and aching, patient compelled to move about for relief. Movement eases pain for a time but patient has to rest and then cycle begins all over again.
Worse: During sleep; cold, wet, rainy weather; after rain; cold bathing; at night; during rest; when lying on back or right side.
Better: Warm, dry weather; motion; walking; change of position; rubbing; warm applications; stretching out limbs.

RUTA

Acts on periosteum and cartilages.
Pains as if bruised.

Bruises of the bone, even old injuries where there is still trouble in the bone will benefit from this remedy.

Lameness after sprains.

Feeling of extreme lassitude, weakness and dispair.

Worse: Lying down; cold, wet weather.

SILICA

Yielding, faint-hearted, anxious.

Lack of grit, moral or physical.

Sensitive to all impressions.

Helps chilly, weak, nervous, timid, shy, faint-hearted people.

Promotes suppuration of boils, abscesses and old wounds that fail to heal.

Expels foreign bodies from the tissues.

Offensive odour from feet, can be caused by suppressed sweat.

Worse: In morning; from washing; uncovering; lying down; lying on left side; damp; cold.

Better: Warmth; wrapping up head; in summer; in wet or humid weather.

STAPHISAGRIA

Very sensitive; violent outbursts; pent up emotions.

A remedy for black eye where there is no relief from cold applications.

Muscles feel bruised, especially of calves.

Extremities feel beaten and painful.

Joints stiff.

Worse: Anger; indignation; grief; least touch on affected part.

Better: Warmth; rest at night.

STRAMONIUM

Loquacity; fears to be alone; wants light and company.

Convulsions of upper extremities and isolated groups of muscles.

Worse: In dark room; when alone; after sleep.

Better: Warmth; in company.

SULPHURIC ACID

Tremors and weakness.

Bad effects of mechanical injuries, with bruises and livid skin.

Worse: Excess of heat or cold; in forenoon and evening.

Better: Warmth and lying on affected side.

SYMPHYTUM

Injuries to sinews, tendons and the periosteum.

Acts on joints generally.

Use for wounds penetrating to perineum and bones and in the non-union of fractures.

Irritable bone at point of fracture.

Pricking pain and soreness of periosteum.

TABACUM

Seasickness with nausea, death-like pallor, icy coldness, and vomiting.

Vertigo on opening eyes.

Terrible faint, sinking feeling at pit of stomach.

Worse: Opening eyes; evening; extremes of heat and cold.

Better: Uncovering; open fresh air.

BOOKS FOR
FURTHER STUDY

HOMOEOPATHY FOR EMERGENCIES by Phyllis Speight.

PERTINENT QUESTIONS AND ANSWERS ABOUT HOMOEOPATHY by Phyllis Speight.

HOMOEOPATHY FOR THE FIRST-AIDER by Dr. Dorothy Shepherd.

HOMOEOPATHY: A GUIDE TO NATURAL MEDICINE by Phyllis Speight.

PUDDEPHATT'S PRIMERS by Noel Puddephatt.

FIRST AID HOMOEOPATHY IN ACCIDENTS AND AILMENTS by Dr. D. M. Gibson.

HOMOEOPATHIC TEACHINGS FROM A MASTER by Edward Cotter.

A STUDY COURSE IN HOMOEOPATHY by Phyllis Speight.

THE ORGANON by Dr. S. Hahnemann.

HOMOEOPATHIC PHARMACIES

Great Britain

Ainsworths Homoeopathic Pharmacy
38 New Cavendish Street
London W1M 7LH (Telephone: 071 935 5330)

Nelsons Homoeopathic Pharmacy
73 Duke Street
Grosvenor Square
London W1M 6BY (Telephone: 081 946 8527)

Galen Homoeopathics
Lewell Mill
West Stafford
Dorchester
Dorset (Telephone: 0305 263996)

Freeman's
7 Eaglesham Road
Clarkston
Glasgow G76 7BU (Telephone: 041 644 1165)

P. A. Janssen
The Pharmacy
28 Ampthill Road
Bedford MK42 9HG (Telephone: 0234 353484)

Jolleys Pharmacy
36 Witton Street
Northwich
Cheshire (Telephone: 0606 331552)

U.S.A.

Boericke & Tafel Inc.
1011 Arch Street
Philadelphia
Pa. 19107

John A. Borneman & Sons
1208 Amosland Road
Norwood
Pa. 19074

Ehrhart & Karl
143 N. Wabash Avenue
Chicago
Ill.

Homoeopathic Educational Services
2124 Kittredge Street
Berkeley
Cal. 94704

Humphreys Pharmacal Inc.
63 Meadow Road 73
Rytherford
New Jersey 07070

Standard Homoeopathic Co.
P.O. Box 61067
Los Angeles
Calif. 90061

Canada

Thompson's Homoeo. Supplies
844 Yonge Street
Toronto
Ont. M4W 2H1

INTRODUCTION TO ACUPRESSURE

In all injuries immediate treatment is desirable and when the appropriate homoeopathic remedy is not at hand Acupressure can be of great help and the treatments that follow have been extracted from *First Aid at Your Finger-Tips* by D. & J. Lawson-Wood. Although Acupuncture and Acupressure have received much publicity during recent years there are many who still doubt its efficacy and it is hoped that the following report by Dr. Alec Forbes M.A., D.M., F.R.C.P., for 28 years consultant physician at Freedomfields Hospital, Plymouth, and co-founder of the Bristol Cancer Help Centre, will induce those in doubt to try this therapy, which has proved effective in numerous instances.

Dr. Forbes wrote:- *I would like to congratulate you and the authors, D. & J. Lawson-Wood, on . . . 'First Aid at Your Finger-Tips'.*

In the two years I have kept the book handy in the car and on holiday it has been used to treat cystitis, cramp, headaches, sunburn, seasickness, pain, hiccoughs and hangover with relief to all these.

Recently I was concerned in a remarkable example of the efficacy of Acupressure. On a skiing holiday in an isolated village without a doctor, two fractures of the leg occurred together. One was a simple fracture of the tibia and fibula with splitting of the tibia. About one hour after the fractures, when the pain was severe, I was able to improve their shock, remove boots and stockings and reduce both fractures and splint them, with the instructor applying pressure on the Kroun-Loun point. I was able to mould the fragments of the second fracture into a passable position as was found when she was admitted to hospital after a two-hour drive down the mountain. Both patients felt no pain during the procedure, although I can vouch for the pain of the second case on the way to hospital, when the Kroun-Loun point was inaccessible. However, I kept the shock under control with the other points.

METHOD OF TREATMENT

For *first-aid* at the points shown on the following pages only the finger-tips or finger-nails need be used. Having located, by reference to the diagram, the exact point to treat, PRESS FIRMLY AND DEEPLY WITH THE TIP OF ONE (OR MORE) FINGER, OR WITH THE FINGER NAIL, the fingers being held at right angles to the flesh. Do not be afraid to dig in quite firmly, even should it hurt a little while being done. In order that the point is *stimulated* there should be a slight rotary or circular boring movement as well as pressure. From half a minute to three or four minutes' treatment will ordinarily suffice.

Unless otherwise indicated *all* the points are bilateral, that is to say, the points are anatomically placed on either side of the body, left and right; moreover, it does not matter on which side the point is treated, nor if both sides are treated together. For example: Severe cramp occurring *anywhere* in the body, muscles or organs, will be treated by applying firm pressure to SING-TSIENN and TRAE-TCHRONG on either the left foot, or the right foot, or on both feet simultaneously.

The reader is reminded that the treatments herein described are for *first-aid* and, though in many instances no other treatment may be needed, in all cases of serious injury or sudden illness, treatment and advice should be obtained as soon as possible from a qualified medical practitioner or other competent person.

There is a very important note to make here; this can be summed up in the expression, "Quantity can sometimes nullify Quality". What we mean to point out by this is simply that just because a "small dose is good, it does NOT follow that a larger dose is better". It seems quite natural to feel that if it is beneficial to massage for two or three minutes it would be even more so to keep it up for twenty or thirty minutes. This line of reasoning does NOT apply when using the Chinese points. Treatment at these points should *never* be carried on for too long — half a minute to four minutes at the most is enough.

The two important factors in this treatment are: First, selecting the correct point to treat; and, second, treating *exactly at that point* for the shortest possible length of time; the whole focus of attention being on *quality* of treatment, not quantity. If you carry on for longer than is necessary you are more likely than not to nullify what you have already done, and your time is wasted without benefit to the patient. Concentrate, therefore, on choosing the correct point; locate it exactly, and then apply a *brief* high quality treatment. It may be found helpful, in order to achieve this, to say under your breath while giving the treatment, "I am treating this point with the intention that . . ." *Have a clear picture in your mind of the result desired, as if it were already achieved.* This is a basic Judo principle.

"I well remember, during a Judo lesson, my instructor had me held firmly down on the mat; for several minutes I struggled in vain, I could not get free. He then asked me, 'What are you trying to do?' 'I'm trying to get out of this hold-down' I answered. Then he said, 'So long as you have a picture of yourself *held down and struggling* you will never get yourself free. Make a picture of yourself *where you want to be*, hold that picture clearly in your mind and then *get into that picture*'. To my joy and surprise, it worked."

ANXIETY

Whenever there is Fear, Restlessness and Anxiety. Chenn-Menn and Tchong-Tchrong.

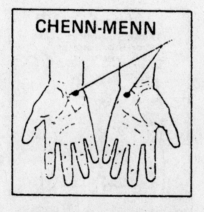

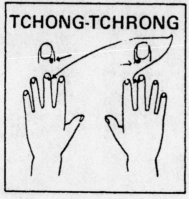

BRUISES

(i) If skin is broken, Iang-Koann.

(ii) If skin is not broken, Tsienn-Iu.

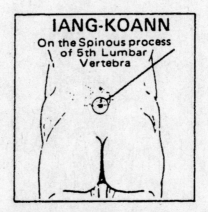

IANG-KOANN

On the Spinous process of 5th Lumbar Vertebra

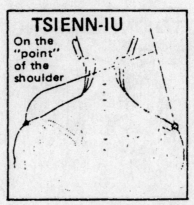

TSIENN-IU

On the "point" of the shoulder

COLD

To raise the body temperature, Tienn-Tsiao.

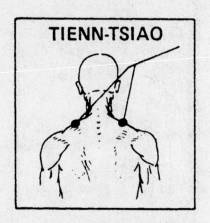

TIENN-TSIAO

COLLAPSE

DEATH SEEMS IMMINENT, Trae-Iuann every half-hour until improvement.

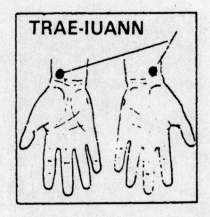

CONCUSSION

(i) For ANY head injury, Tsienn-Iu.
(ii) If death seems imminent, Trae-Iuann.

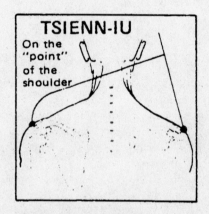

TSIENN-IU

On the "point" of the shoulder

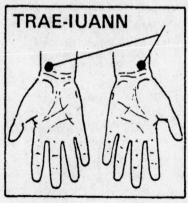

TRAE-IUANN

(iii) If caused by spinal injury, Iang-Koann.

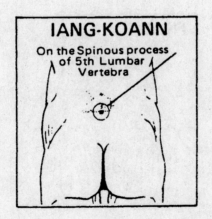

(iv) If blood is oozing from ears and mouth, Chang-Tsiao and Tchao-Rae left side followed in ten minutes by Tsienn-Iu.

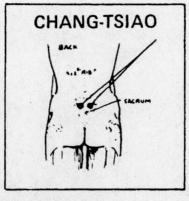

CHANG-TSIAO

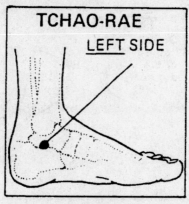

TCHAO-RAE

LEFT SIDE

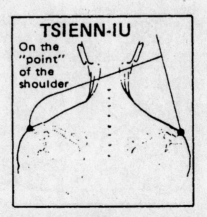

TSIENN-IU

On the "point" of the shoulder

CRAMP

FOR ALL CRAMPS AND SPASMS

Sing-Tsienn and Trae-Tchrong

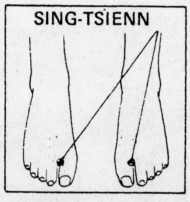

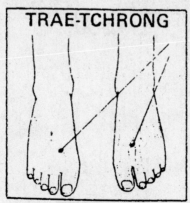

FOR ACUTE STRICTURE (Painful retention of urine) Add Li-Keou.

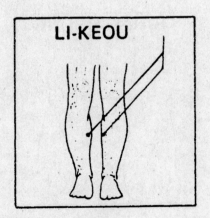

LI-KEOU

EXHAUSTION

(i) Physical, Tchong-Tchou.
(ii) Nervous and Mental, Chao-Rae.

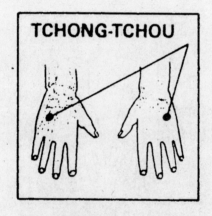

TCHONG-TCHOU

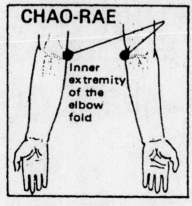

CHAO-RAE

Inner extremity of the elbow fold

FAINTING

(i) If from fear and apprehension, Chenn-Menn.

(ii) If there are any hysterical symptoms, Oe-Ling.

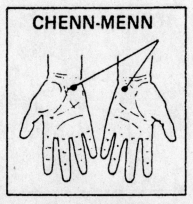

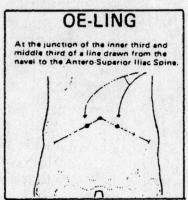

(iii) Heart failure: severe pain over the heart radiating to left arm feeling as if chest is in a vice. Followed by cold sweat and collapse, Tienn-Tchre or Ta-Ling.

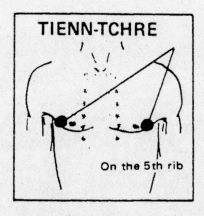

TIENN-TCHRE

On the 5th rib

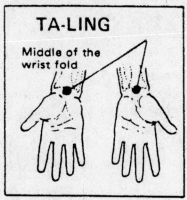

TA-LING

Middle of the wrist fold

FATIGUE

For the effects arising from excessive fatigue,
Tsienn-Iu.

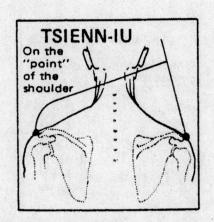

FRACTURES and SPRAINS

(i) If skin is bruised, broken, crushed, etc., to relieve the pain, Kroun-Loun and/or Iang-Koann.

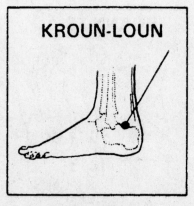

KROUN-LOUN

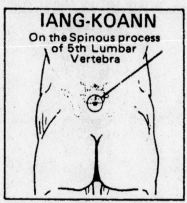

IANG-KOANN
On the Spinous process
of 5th Lumbar
Vertebra

(ii) For sprains in general, Roann-Tsiao.
(iii) In fractures, after the bone has been set use Ta-Tchrou to assist healing of the break.

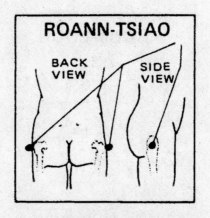

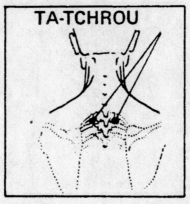

SPRAINS IN GENERAL

Tchong-Tsi and/or Roann-Tsiao.

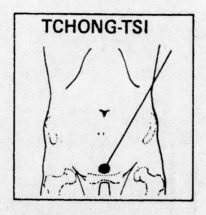

TCHONG-TSI

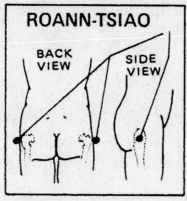

ROANN-TSIAO

BACK VIEW

SIDE VIEW

HEAD INJURY

For all head injuries whether slight or severe;
Tsienn-Iu.

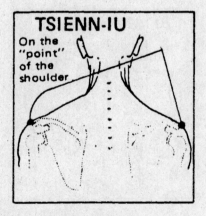

WOUNDS, CUTS, BRUISES, etc.

(i) If bruised and crushed, Tsienn-Iu.
(ii) If lacerated, torn, Iang-Koann.

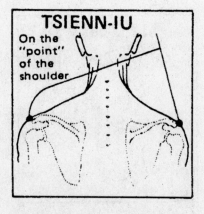

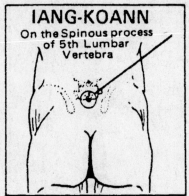

(iii) Punctures and deep cuts, Ledum.
(iv) Severely torn wounds, grazes, Iang-Koann.
(v) Crushed fingernail, Iang-Koann.

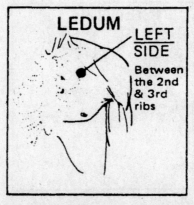

LEDUM

LEFT SIDE

Between the 2nd & 3rd ribs

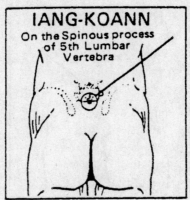

IANG-KOANN

On the Spinous process of 5th Lumbar Vertebra

TETANUS

(i) To prevent tetanus treat immediately Ledum.
(ii) If there is twitching of muscles *round the wound only*, Iang-Koann.

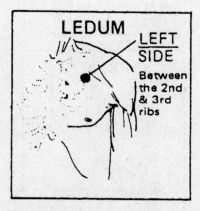

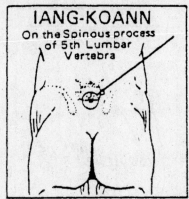

(iii) Where slightest touch aggravates spasms. Li-Toe and/or Chou-Kou and/or Inn-Ling-Tsiuann (left).

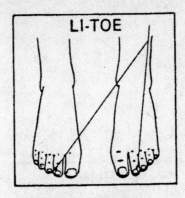

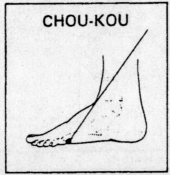

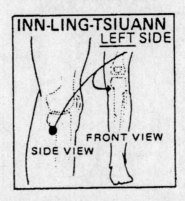

LOCATION OF POINTS

CHANG-TSIAO

When a person is standing upright there are two dimples, one either side of the spine, above the buttocks, on the lower part of the waist line. When the person bends forwards, instead of dimples there are bony prominences. The first sacral foramen is halfway between a dimple (or bony prominence) and the mid line of the spine.

CHAO-RAE

Exactly at the inner extremity of the elbow fold.

CHENN-MENN

On the wrist fold, little finger side, close to the small pea shaped bone (the pisiform) where the ulna artery can be felt. This is about a finger's width from the end of the wrist fold.

CHOU-KOU

Near the base of the little toe, just behind the prominence that is felt at the end of the metatarsal bone at the little toe joint.

IANG-KOANN

On the spinous process of the last lumbar vertebra, **not** on its tip but near the dip between the processes of the fourth and fifth vertebrae.

INN-LING-TSIUANN

Left side. On the leg below the knee joint in the little hollow felt under the head of the Tibia (bone).

KROUN-LOUN

Between the outer ankle and Achilles tendon, press down on to the heel bone.

LEDUM

This is not a Chinese acupuncture point. It was discovered by Dr. Weihe as corresponding in its action with the homoeopathic remedy in potency Ledum Palustra. As a first-aid remedy Dr. Dorothy Mazel recommended an immediate dose of Ledum if there is **any** risk of tetanus. The point is reached by going up into the armpit to the second intercostal space. Between the second and third ribs.

LI-KEOU

Draw a line on the inner side of the leg from the ankle to the level of the knee-cap. Divide the line into fifteen equal parts. The point is six fifteenths up from the inner ankle.

LI-TOE
At the outer angle of the root of the second toenail.

OE-LING
Drawings show position clearly.

ROANN-TSIAO
Drawings show position clearly.

SING-TSIENN
Drawings show position clearly.

TA-LING
In the middle of the wrist fold.

TA-TCHROU
Drawings show position clearly.

TCHAO-RAE
One finger's width vertically below the most prominent point of the inner ankle bone.

TCHONG-TCHOU
Drawings show position clearly.

TCHONG-TCHRONG
Drawings show position clearly.

TCHONG-TSI
Drawings show position clearly.

TIENN-TCHRE
On males the point is in the fourth intercostal space one finger's width beyond the outer edge of the nipple areola. In females the point will be correspondingly in the fourth intercostal space.

TIENN-TSIAO
On the shoulder muscle (trapezius) halfway between the mid-line of the back of the neck and the point of the shoulder.

TRAE-IUANN
Outer extremity of the wrist fold thumb side. This point is also known as 'The corpse reviver'.

TRAE-TCHRONG
Drawings show position clearly.

TSIENN-IU
On 'point' of the shoulder.